Cooking My Way

For Christmas Day

From Sunrise to Sunset
Cheap Nutritious Food

Helen Thomas

First published 2017

Publisher: Grubooks

Email: orders@grubooks.com

© Helen Thomas 2017

Email: helen@wise.works

The moral rights of the author have been asserted

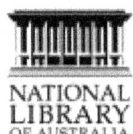 A catalogue record for this book is available from the National Library of Australia

Creator: Thomas, Helen, 1946- author
       Thomas, Hilton, 1943- also contributed.

Title: Cooking my way for Christmas day: from sunrise to sunset - cheap nutritious food / Helen Thomas.

ISBN: 9781925319071 (paperback)

ISBN 9781925319088 (Epub)

Subjects: Low budget cooking.
Cooking.
Nutrition.

All rights reserved. Except as permitted under the *Australian Copyright Act* 1968 (for example a fair dealing for the purposes of study, research, criticism or review), no part of this book may be reproduced, stored in a retrieval system, communicated, or transmitted in any form or by any means without prior written permission. All enquiries should be made to the publisher at the address above.

Disclaimer

The material in this book is of the nature of general information only. The information in this book is not intended to be taken as medical advice or to indicate the suitability of particular foods in any specific circumstances. The publisher and author expressly disclaim any liability to any person because of any action taken or not taken in reliance, in whole or in part, on the content of this publication. If you have medical issues, you should consult a qualified medical practitioner.

Contents

Introduction iv

Starters/Entrées 2
    Goats Cheese 2
    Prawn Cocktail 2
    Asparagus in salmon 2

Meat Dishes 3
    Roast Turkey 4
    Hilton's Marinated Lamb 6
    Stuffed Roast Pork 8
    Baked Ham 10

Vegetables 11
    Roast Potatoes 12
    Steamed Broccoli and Carrots 13
    Roast Mixed Vegetables 14

Sauces 15
    Roast Vegetable Gravy 16
    Parsnip Puree 17
    Red-currant sauce 18

Desserts 19
    Pavlova 20
    Fruit Salad with Ice Cream 21
    Christmas Pudding with Brandy Butter 22
    Iced Coffee 23

Leftovers 25
    Turkey Patties 26
    Lamb Kebabs 27
    Pork stir-fry 28
    Ham and Egg Cauliflower Bake 29

Introduction

Dear Readers

Christmas will soon be upon us, and many of us are going to be wondering what to have for Christmas day, and how we are going to be able to afford it.

Let me tell you how my husband, Hilton, and I do it. We have a lovely day on Christmas day. We have ten to 12 people around the table for Christmas lunch.

We live in Australia. Food and the cost of living are expensive, and we are on pensions, so we have to be careful with our money.

We start planning and costing in November. We write down what we hope to give our guests and then make a list of the food we intend to buy.

We start with the starters/entrées. We have had different starters/entrées. Here are some suggestions to choose from:

- Asparagus rolled in salmon with a cherry tomato on a slice of pumpernickel bread.
- Prawn Cocktail: Prawns on a bed of lettuce with a tomato and seafood cocktail sauce.
- A slice of toasted bread with goat's cheese, slices of red, green, and yellow peppers, cherry tomatoes, and lettuce leaves

Then for the main course, we have

- Roast turkey.
- A piece of pork with crackling.
- A piece of ham.
- We buy a joint of lamb and marinate it for a week in different spices. I will tell you how we cook it.

These are accompanied by:

- Roast potatoes sprinkled with mixed herbs and a dash of salt,
- steamed baby carrots and steamed Brussels sprouts.
- Parsnip Puree. (Hilton makes this. It is really tasty and easy to make).
- Gravy (Again, Hilton makes a delicious gravy with the meat juices.)
- Salad,
- A large tray of diced mixed vegetables roasted with a dash of oil and herbs.

Our friends and family help by bringing a dish. I discuss with them what they intend to bring towards the meal.

For dessert, I talk to our guests and find out if they can bring one dessert. One of my guests may be keen to bring a pavlova and decorate it, another may wish to bring a bowl of fruit salad, and I may be able to buy a large container of ice cream (vanilla goes well with almost everything), and some pouring cream. If another of my guests offers to bring a dessert, I would ask them to bring a Christmas pudding.

So we have a pavlova, a bowl of fruit salad and ice cream, and a Christmas pudding with pouring cream. Let me tell you, dear readers, my guests are so pleased that I asked them to be part of the day's expense. After all, all the good feeling on Christmas should come from the heart in the form of giving.

Have a lovely Christmas, and we wish you and your family and friends all the very best in the coming years. I will be keeping up with my cookery books.

Cheers
Helen Thomas

The recipes in this book will generally result in generous quantities of food. I prefer to provide more than will be eaten on the day and then freeze and reuse leftovers.

Food that has been defrosted should not be refrozen unless it has been cooked.

You need to avoid having food kept at room temperature for long periods of time. If you have cooked meat left over, try to freeze it as soon as you can. See page 25 for recipes for delicious ways of using leftovers.

Starters/Entrées

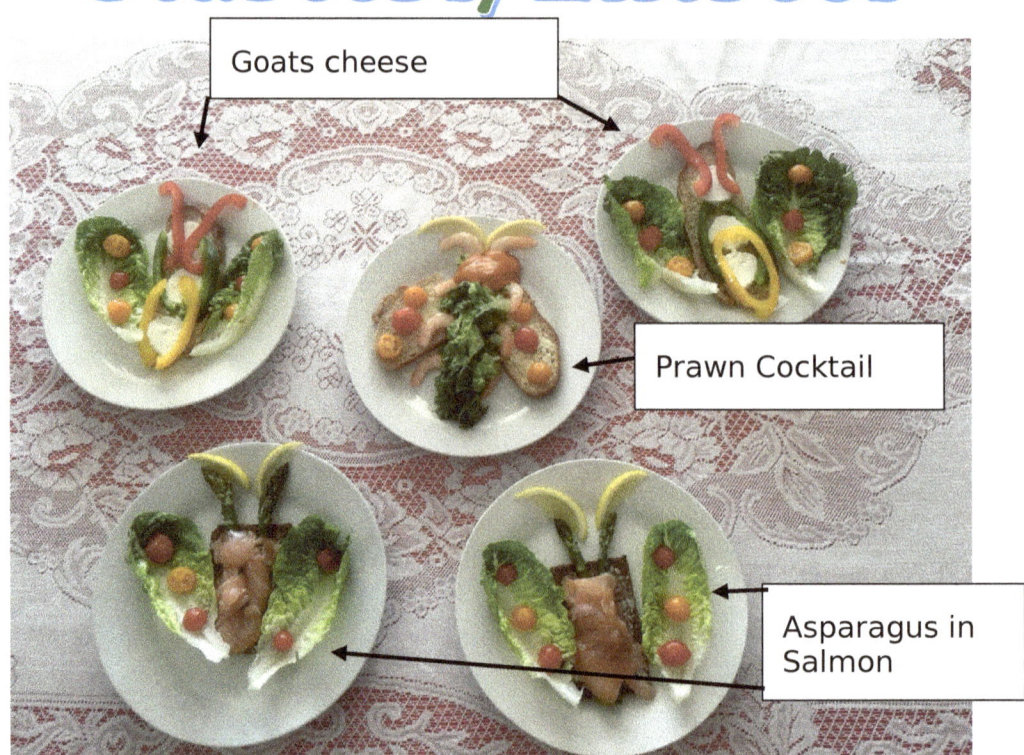

When preparing starters, I always concentrate on presentation. It is said that we eat first with our eyes, then with our nose, and lastly with our mouth. The appearance of food is important, so I use contrasting colours and a beautiful arrangement on the plate. I don't provide too much for a starter. It is just a preparation for the meal, and I don't want to fill our guests up before the main course!

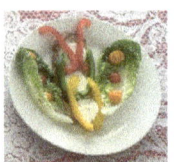
Goats Cheese

A slice of rye bread, lightly toasted, with two or three rounds of goats' cheese, a slice of green pepper, a slice of red pepper, cherry tomatoes and lettuce leaves.

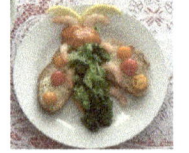
Prawn Cocktail

In a small bowl, arrange two lettuce leaves (washed thoroughly), on the bottom of the bowl. Arrange cooked and shelled prawns around the bowl on the lettuce. Pour a bit of Seafood Cocktail Sauce to taste. Add a dash of salt and pepper. You can serve this with a small wedge of lemon.

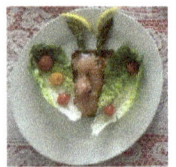
Asparagus in salmon

Use 2 Asparagus spears per person. Use nice plump dark green spears. The Asparagus has to be steamed but don't over-steam them, or they will break up. Take a slice of smoked salmon and roll the asparagus in the salmon. Serve it on a slice of pumpernickel bread with cherry tomatoes for decoration.

Meat Dishes

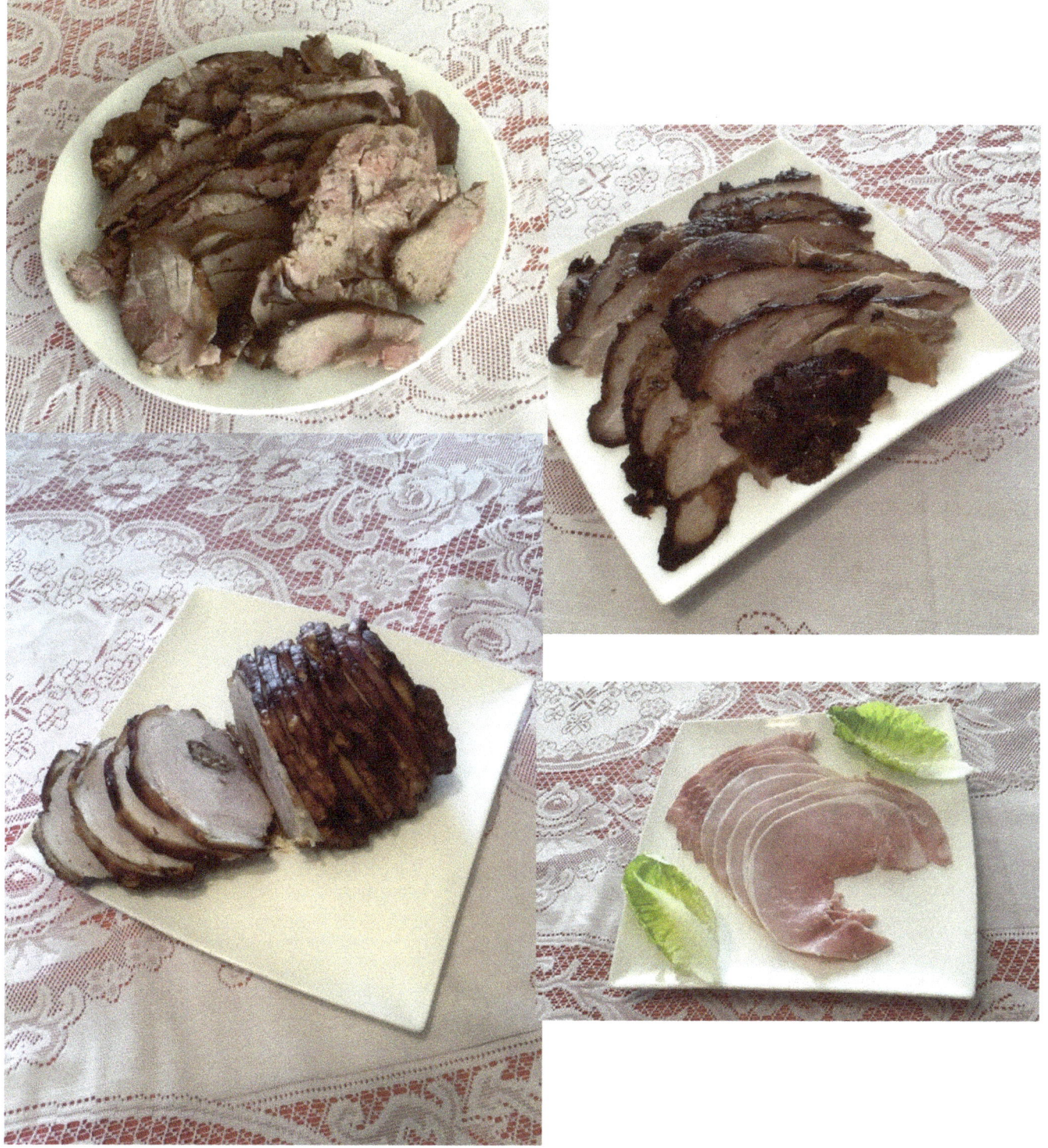

Roast Turkey

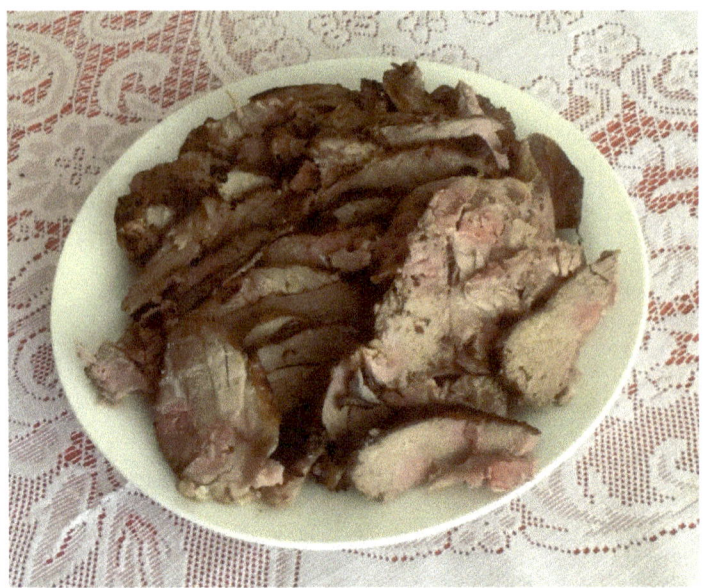

Ingredients

1 Turkey (size depends on number of people)

3 or more slices stale bread

1 onion

8 rashers bacon

Ginger paste

Garlic paste

Mixed herbs

Salt and Pepper

1 egg

Dijon mustard

Balsamic vinegar

Method

The turkey should be completely thawed. Take out the giblets from the cavity. If you are making your own stuffing follow this method:

Stuffing

Depending on the size of the cavity, break up 3 or more slices of stale bread.

Chop an onion.

Cut the rind off 4 rashers of bacon and cut the rashers into small squares.

Mix all together.

Add a dash of ginger paste and garlic paste.

Add a generous amount of mixed herbs.

Season to taste with salt and pepper.

Mix an egg into the mixture to bind it.

Fill the cavity with the mixture. Push the mixture into the cavity as far as it will go.

I usually sew the cavity together with a large darning needle and string.

Cooking the turkey

Pat the turkey dry with kitchen paper. Sprinkle with salt.

Make a paste in a bowl with Dijon mustard, a dash of ginger paste and garlic paste, and a dash of balsamic vinegar.

Rub the paste all over the turkey. This paste really helps the turkey not to dry up and gives it a lovely taste.

Make sure the oven is hot. 220°C (430°F) Cook at this heat for first 30 Minutes.

Turn temperature down to 200°C (390°F)

After another hour, take the turkey out and cover it with rashers of bacon. Baste the turkey thoroughly with the juices several times during the cooking.

Stick a meat thermometer into the middle of the turkey meat. Make sure it is cooked properly and the thermometer reads 190°C (375°F).

You need to keep an eye on the turkey while it is cooking, baste frequently to make sure it does not get dry.

When the turkey is cooked, put it on the serving plate and save the juices and residue in the baking tin for the gravy. (See gravy recipes on page 16)

Tips

When working out meat quantities allow 125 to 250 grams (4 to 8 ounces) of meat per person or more because we all like to be greedy at Christmas. This is the total meat for one meal so if you have four kinds of meat you will need less of each.

Eat slowly, so you enjoy your food.

Remember your portion control

Hilton's Marinated Lamb

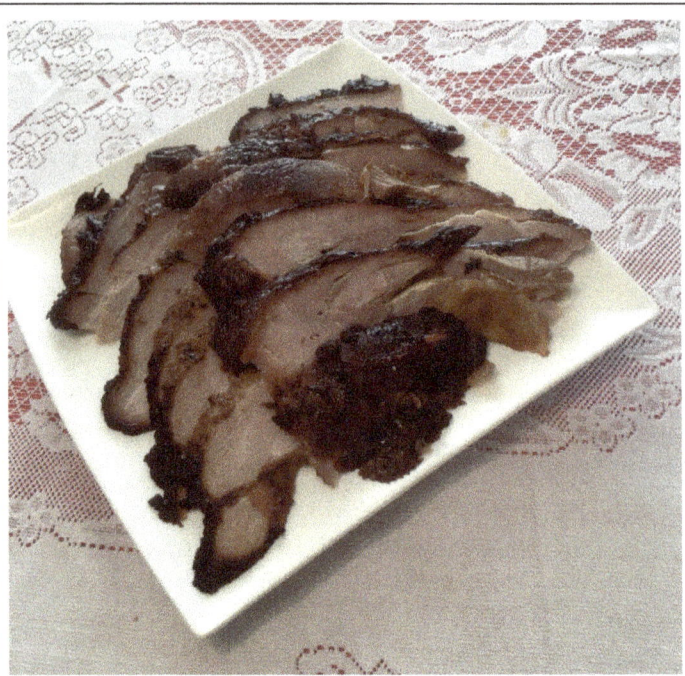

Ingredients

Leg or shoulder of lamb

4 cloves garlic

2 rashers bacon

For Marinade

1 Onion

2-3 cloves garlic

1 tsp coarse salt

3 sticks celery

1 carrot

1 Tbsp mixed herbs

1 tbsp Rosemary

10 Juniper berries (crushed)

4 bay leaves

1 tsp whole black peppercorns

1 cup oil

½ cup white wine vinegar

½ cup white wine

Method

Chop all vegetables

Cook onion in oil until transparent

Add other vegetables and brown them lightly

Add vinegar and wine and simmer until vegetables are soft.

Add herbs spices, salt, and peppercorns

Continue simmering for a few minutes

Allow to cool completely

Remove skin and surplus fat from lamb, trying not to damage the meat

Pierce holes in the meat with a sharp, narrow knife and insert small strips of bacon and slivers of garlic

Put the lamb in a large snaplock bag and cover with the cooled marinade. Squeeze out the air and seal.

Keep in fridge for 3 days turning at least once per day.

Remove the lamb from the bag. Scrape off all the marinade and vegetables, Dry with kitchen paper.

Put in a roasting pan, on a rack and pour oil over

Heat oven to 240°C (465°F) and cook for 30 minutes. Turn oven down to 180°C (360°F) and continue cooking for a further 1 hour per kilo, (25 minutes per pound) basting frequently.

When the meat is cooked (it will start drawing back from the bones. You can use a meat thermometer to check) remove it from the oven, cover and allow it to rest for 20 minutes before carving.

Use the meat juices to make gravy (recipes on page 16), You can add red-currant jelly to the gravy or serve red-currant jelly separately if available.

Tips

Eat slowly, so you enjoy your food.

Remember your portion control

Stuffed Roast Pork

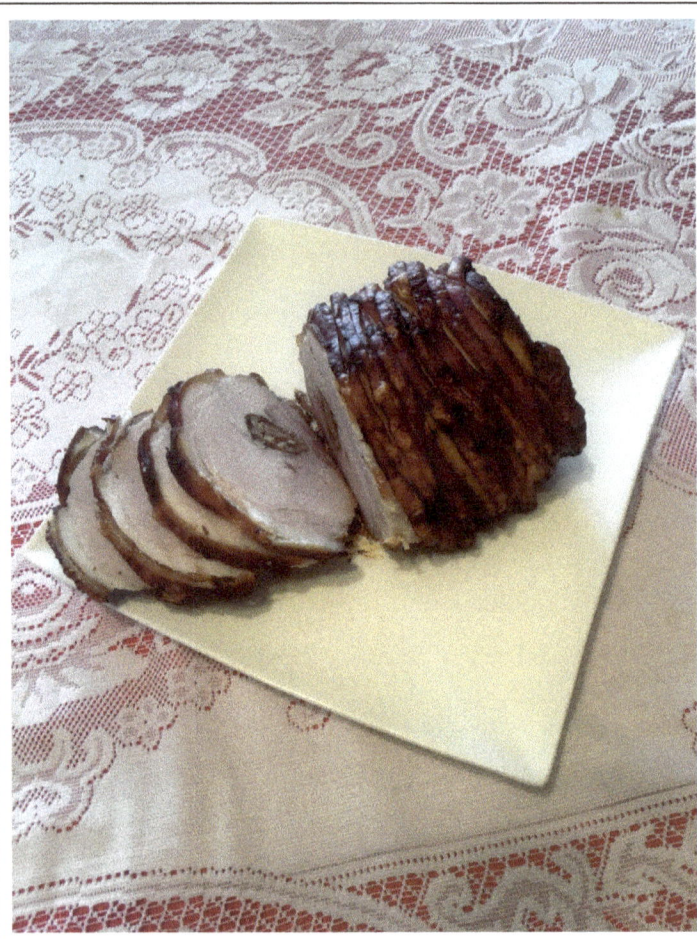

Ingredients

Boneless rolled leg of pork
Mustard
Ginger paste
Garlic paste
Salt
Pepper
Oil

<u>For stuffing</u>
1 onion chopped
Breadcrumbs or fine oatmeal
6 Prunes
1 chopped apple
1 egg
Tsp mixed herbs
½ Tsp ground coriander
½ Tsp Garlic paste
½ Tsp Ginger paste
Salt and pepper

Method

I buy boneless rolled pork leg. Currently, in Australia, this is one of the cheapest meats. However, I do not use it as it is prepared by the shop.

First, remove the string or net bag holding it together and then unroll it. Take some of the meat out of the middle – this is often loose pieces of meat. Take out about ⅓ of the meat, dice it and keep it in the freezer for another meal.

Rub the meat with a mixture of mustard, ginger, garlic, salt and pepper.

Make some more cuts in the skin, so it has a cut every ¼ inch (6 mm). I find a Stanley knife is the best for this, but be careful! The cuts should just go through the skin into the fat, not right through to the meat.

Make the stuffing by mixing together the stuffing ingredients.

Put this mixture in the meat and roll it up again. If the meat was held together by an elastic net, reuse this. Otherwise, tie it up with kitchen twine making sure to tie the ends tightly, to hold the stuffing in.

Thoroughly dry the skin with kitchen paper and rub it with salt and oil.

Roast this in a preheated oven at 240°C (465°F) for 30 minutes to set the crackling, then lower the oven to 200 and cook for 80 minutes per kilo (35 minutes per pound) and check it is cooked with a meat thermometer.

Finish the crackling off with 15 minutes in a hot oven 240°C (465°F).

My friends love crackling, so I try to make sure it is well done and crisp, but not burned.

Tips

Eat slowly, so you enjoy your food.

Remember your portion control

Baked Ham

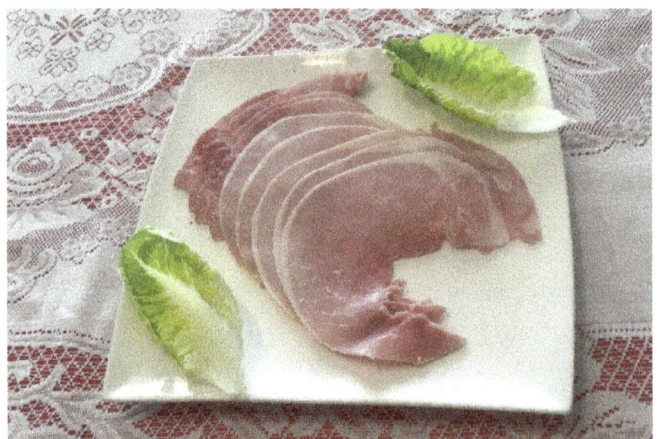

Ingredients

Leg or half leg smoked ham

About 40 cloves

Mustard

Honey

Lemon Juice

Method

Sometimes I buy sliced ham off the bone (shown in photo), but if there are many people coming, and I want to make it more showy, I do baked ham.

Remove the skin from the ham, trying to leave the fat in place. Sometimes it is easy to do, but you may need to cut the skin in strips with a very sharp knife, being careful not to cut into the fat more than necessary. Then pull the strips of skin off.

Cut into the fat, not cutting into the meat, making a diamond pattern with diagonal cuts both ways about 1 cm (1/2 inch) apart.

Rub the lamb with a mixture of mustard, honey, and lemon Juice. Put a clove in the centre of each diamond of fat, piercing through to the meat.

Bake the ham in the oven for about 2 hours on a low heat 180°C (360°F), basting a few times. The fat should shrink showing up the diamond pattern and get a golden colour from the caramelised honey. This way of preparing ham looks quite dramatic if it is served whole and carved at the table, as well as being delicious.

Tips

Eat slowly, so you enjoy your food.

Remember your portion control

Vegetables

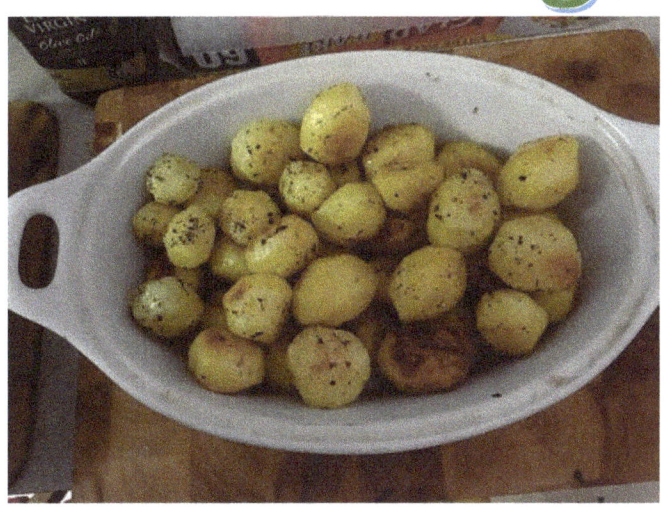

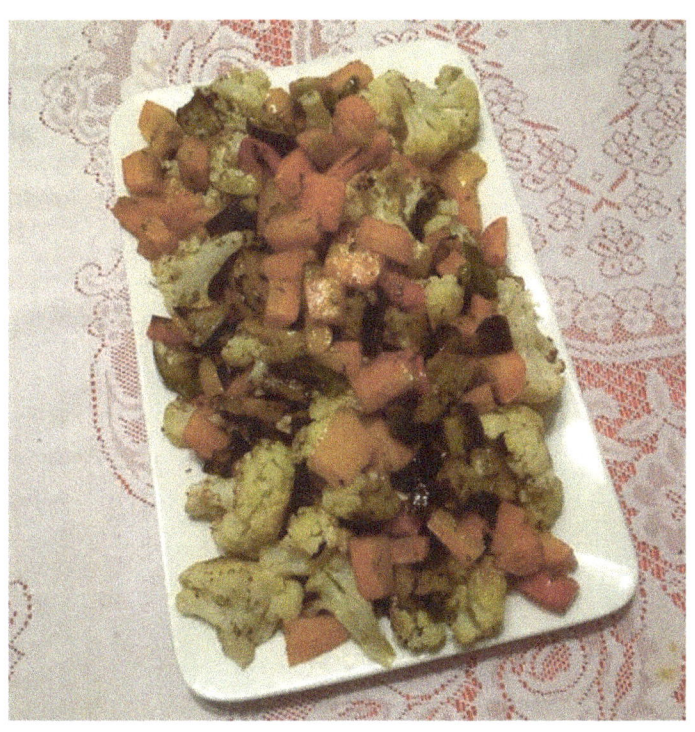

Roast Potatoes

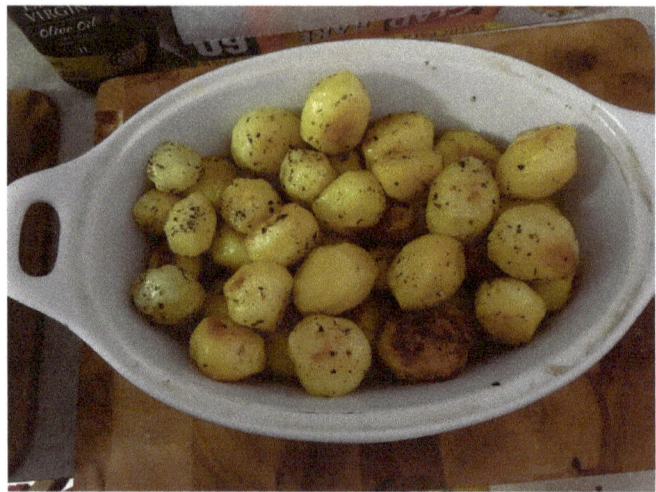

Ingredients

Small potatoes
Oil
Mixed herbs
Salt

Method

Preheat oven to 200°C (395°F)

Peel the potatoes. If there is a lot of variation in size cut the larger ones in half

Boil potatoes for 15 minutes in salted water and drain

Put in a roasting tin with some oil

Sprinkle with mixed herbs and salt

Roast for 45 minutes to an hour, basting 2 or 3 times, until they are a rich brown.

Tips

Eat slowly, so you enjoy your food.
Remember your portion control

Steamed Broccoli and Carrots

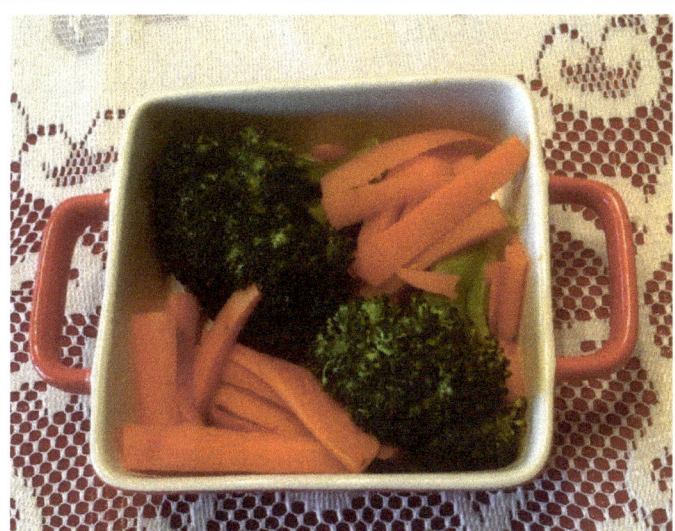

Ingredients

You can use any vegetables you want. In the photo, I have used broccoli florets and julienned carrots.

Other ideas you may like try include:

- Brussels Sprouts (perhaps with Cashew nuts)
- Runner beans or French beans
- Sugar snap peas

Method

The idea is to give an easy to eat, easy to prepare, nutritious and delicious vegetable.

Pay attention to colour and appearance as well. The look of the food makes a huge difference to how we feel about it.

You may be able to jazz up the vegetable with some nuts, herbs, spices, etc.

The steaming process is simply putting the vegetables in a colander over a pan of boiling water, and covering with a lid to trap the steam.

Hard vegetables such as carrot may need to be steamed a bit longer than soft vegetables like the broccoli.

Tips

Do not throw the broccoli stalks away. They can be used in the gravy or used later in a stir-fry. The carrot peelings can also be used in the gravy if the carrots were well washed before peeling.

Eat slowly, so you enjoy your food.

Remember your portion control

Roast Mixed Vegetables

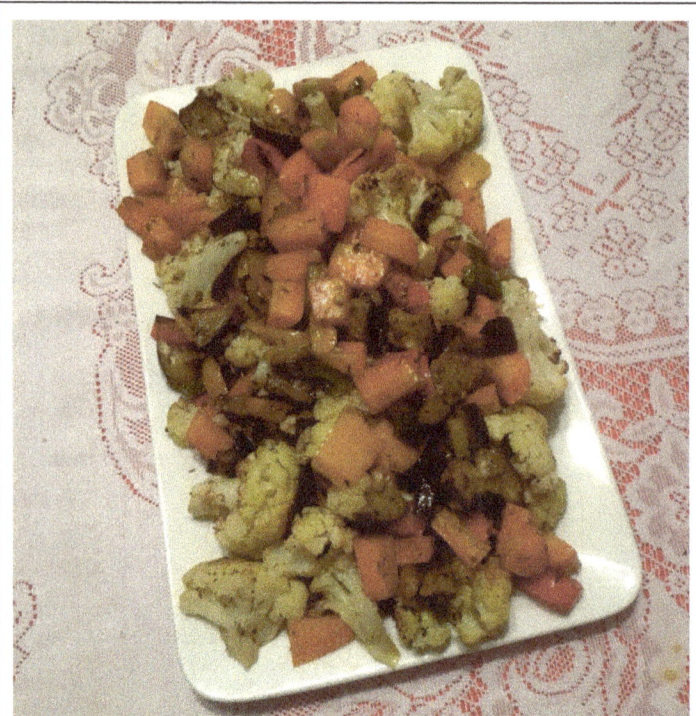

Ingredients

Use several different vegetables, aiming for different colours and textures as well as different tastes. This makes the dish interesting, beautiful and appetising as well as being healthy.

I typically use pumpkin, cauliflower, broccoli, eggplant (aubergine), carrots, and peppers. You can also include others depending on what is available.

Mixed dried herbs.

Salt to taste

Method

Wash all the vegetables.

Peel as required

Cut the vegetables up into convenient pieces. Aim for similar sizes.

With hard vegetables such as pumpkin and carrots, par-boil them before roasting.

Line an oven tray with foil and put a little cooking oil on it. Spread it to grease the foil and reduce sticking.

Put all the vegetables on the foil, spreading them out as much as possible.

Sprinkle with oil, mixed dried herbs and a little salt.

Bake in a moderate oven (180°C 360°F) for about 30 minutes until they start browning on top.

Tips

Eat slowly, so you enjoy your food.

Remember your portion control

Sauces

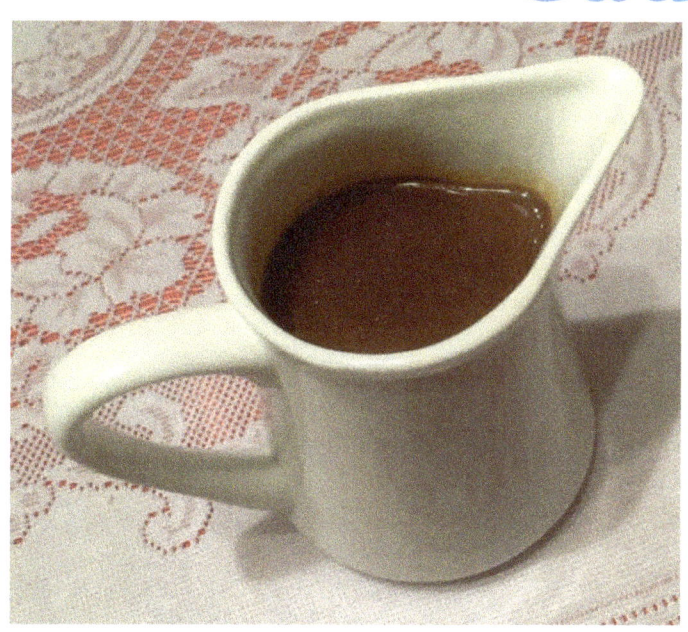

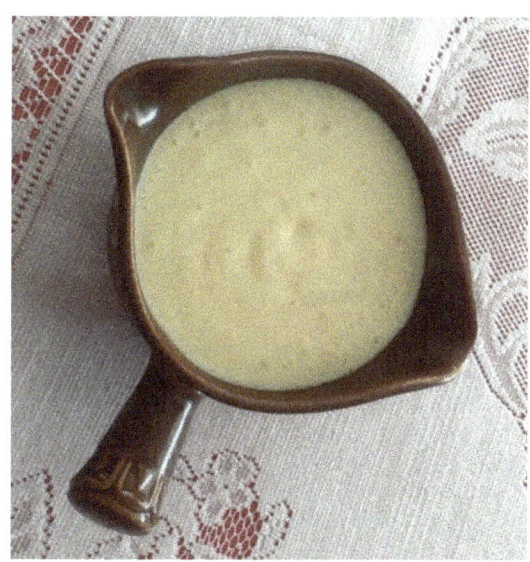

Roast Vegetable Gravy

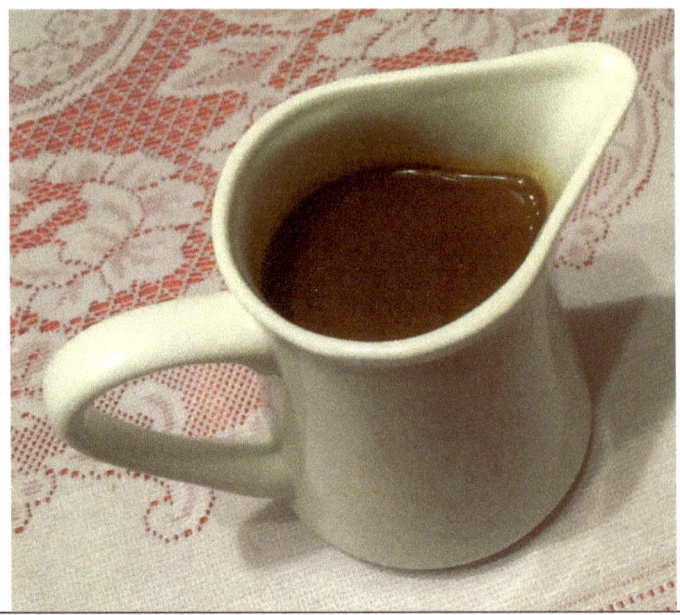

Ingredients

Fat and pan scrapings from roasting meat

Onion

Garlic or garlic paste

Vegetable peelings (see method)

1 tsp Sugar

Vegetable water

Stock

Oyster sauce/soy sauce/ Worcestershire sauce (Optional)

Salt and Pepper

Method

Start with the fat from roasting the meat, scrape it with all the bits in the roasting pan into a saucepan. Over a moderate heat add a chopped onion, some chopped garlic and fry these in the fat until the onion is transparent. Then add any vegetable peelings, well washed (not potato peel). These would typically include the outer leaves of sprouts, cabbage, even lettuce; bean ends, carrot and parsnip peel. Mushroom stalks and peel are also excellent. If there is not much in the way of vegetable peelings you may need to chop some vegetables. Fry these until browned slightly. Then add some sugar on the bottom of the pan. Let the sugar melt and caramelise a bit then stir it with the vegetables.

Add some vegetable water, and/or stock, bring to the boil and simmer for 10 minutes.

Strain and force as much of the vegetables as possible through a fine wire sieve, or liquidise in a blender. Add more stock if it is too thick. Add sauces if desired.

Taste and season as required. Don't add too much salt as there will have been salt in the added liquids.

Tips

This is gluten-free if you use gluten-free stock and sauces or don't add these.

Eat slowly, so you enjoy your food.

Remember your portion control

Parsnip Puree

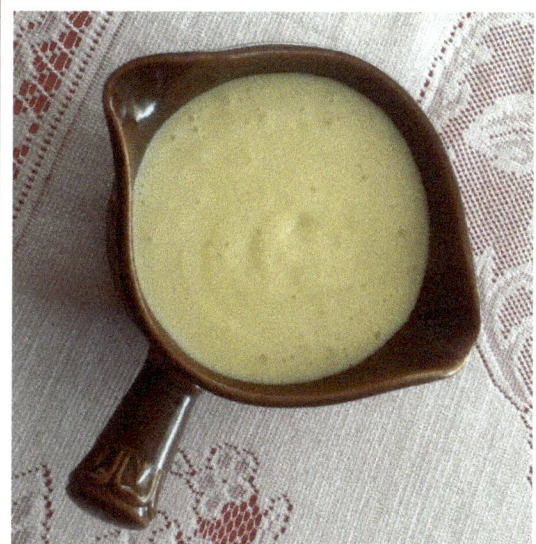

Ingredients

½ kilo (1 lb) parsnips

4 cloves garlic

½ cup double cream

¼ cup butter

1 cup milk

Method

Peel and chop the parsnips.

Put all ingredients in a saucepan with a lid over a medium heat.

Bring nearly to a boil and simmer for 10-15 minutes until the parsnips are very soft.

Remove lid and continue cooking for further 5 minutes to reduce liquid.

Put in a blender and then strain through a fine sieve.

Bring back to heat, taste, and season to taste.

Tips

Eat slowly, so you enjoy your food.

Remember your portion control

Redcurrant sauce

Ingredients

1 small Onion
½ tsp Garlic
Oil
1 glass red wine
½ glass brandy
½ cup redcurrant jelly
I tbsp cornflour
1 cup chicken or vegetable stock
Salt and pepper to taste

Method

Melt the chopped onion in a little oil
Add the garlic and fry for one minute
Add the red wine and brandy, Bring to the boil
Stir in the redcurrant jelly
Mix the cornflour with the stock
Add to the mixture and bring to the boil.
Boil for a minute stirring well until it thickens
Taste and season
Strain through a fine wire sieve.

Tips

This is excellent with strong meat, e.g. turkey, lamb, or venison
Eat slowly, so you enjoy your food.
Remember your portion control

Desserts

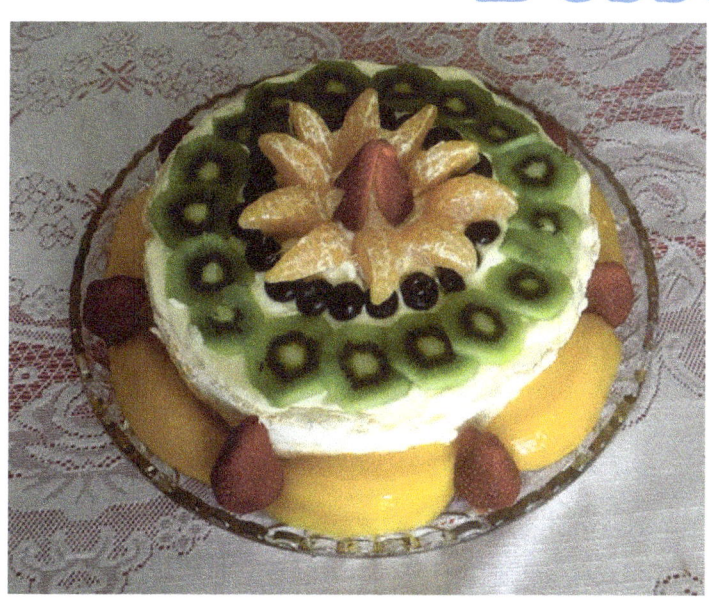

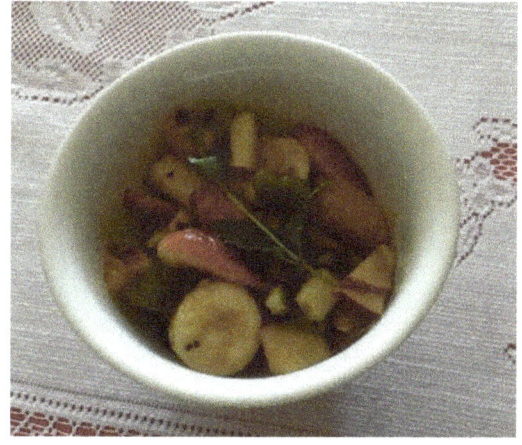

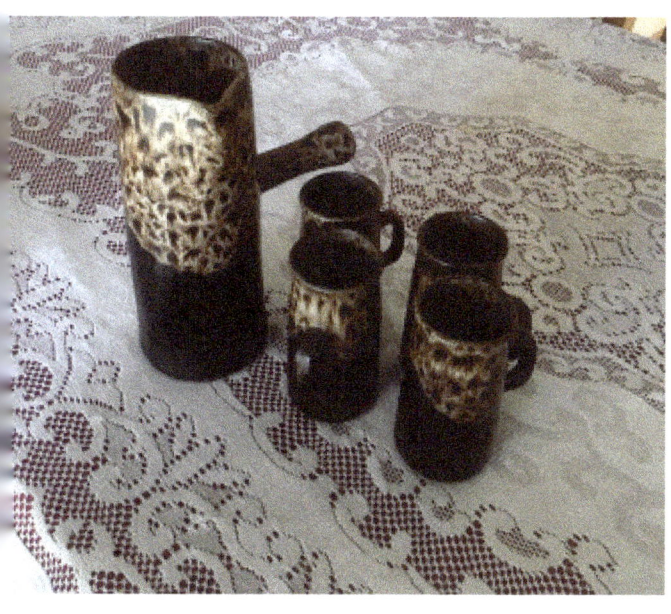

Pavlova

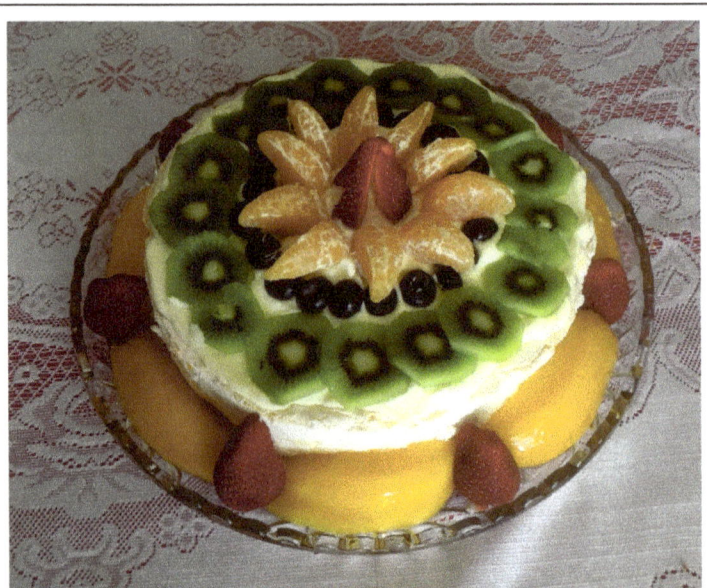

Ingredients

1 Bought pavlova base. I usually buy a large one.

2 cups thickened or double cream

½ cup caster sugar

A few drops vanilla essence

Fruit of your choice

Method

Beat cream until it starts to thicken.

Add sugar and vanilla. Continue beating until it becomes stiff enough to form peaks. <u>Don't over beat it or it will turn to butter!!</u>

Spread cream onto the top and sides of the pavlova. It will tend to run down a bit at the edges but don't worry. You can use fruit to cover this up as I have done in the photo. You do not need to get it perfect as it will be mostly covered with fruit.

Decorate it with fruit of your choice.

Keep in refrigerator until you are ready to serve it or the cream may become too runny.

Tips

Eat slowly, so you enjoy your food.

Remember your portion control

Fruit Salad with Ice Cream

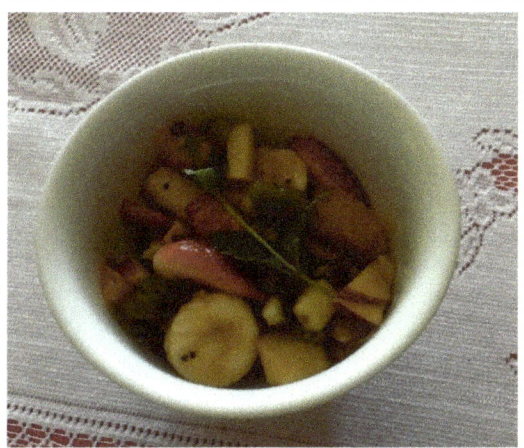

Ingredients

A variety of fresh or tinned fruit depending on what is available. We used

Apple

Banana

Strawberries

Kiwifruit

Mandarin

Pineapple

Sugar

Mint leaves

Method

Cut the fruit up and mix together.

Sprinkle with sugar – coconut sugar is good for this

Cover with a plate and weight it down with a couple of tins or something.

Leave in refrigerator for 24 hours

Stir in a few chopped mint leaves (optional)

Decorate with mint sprigs

Tips

Serve with ice cream and/or whipped cream.

Eat slowly, so you enjoy your food.

Remember your portion control

Christmas Pudding with Brandy Butter

Ingredients

Christmas pudding

<u>For brandy butter</u>

1 cup unsalted butter

1 cup caster sugar or icing sugar

2 tbsp brandy

Method

I generally buy a Christmas pudding. It is not worth the effort of making it.

You can heat it in a microwave or steam it according to the instructions.

You can serve it with pouring cream or custard, but brandy butter makes it a bit more special

<u>To make Brandy Butter</u>

The butter must be at a warm room temperature – not difficult while Christmas cooking is going on – so it is very soft but not melted.

Mix the butter with the sugar to make a smooth paste.

Stir in the brandy until the colour is consistent

Put into a bowl and mark the top with a fork to make it pretty

Keep in a refrigerator for at least an hour to stiffen before serving.

Tips

Eat slowly, so you enjoy your food.

Remember your portion control

Iced Coffee

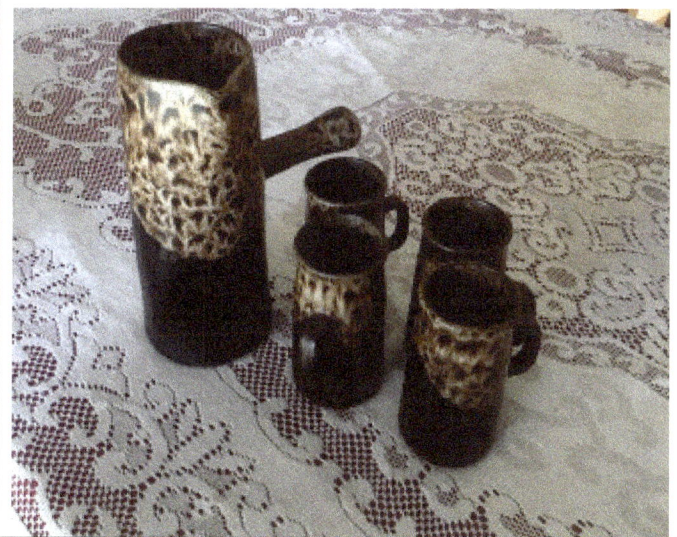

Ingredients

½ litre (1 pt) water

6 tsp coffee extract or instant coffee

1 cup condensed milk

½ tsp vanilla essence

Method

Boil the water and add the coffee. Add the condensed milk and vanilla

Stir well

Refrigerate

Serve cold

Tips

Eat slowly, so you enjoy your food.

Remember your portion control

Leftovers

Turkey

If you have turkey leftover from Christmas Lunch, cut it up into small pieces, put in freezer bags, and freeze. Allow enough turkey in each bag to make Turkey Patties

Lamb

If you have leftover lamb, I suggest that you can make Lamb Kebabs.

Pork

Leftover pork makes an excellent Pork Stir-Fry that is quick and easy to make.

Ham

With leftover ham, try my very tasty Ham and Egg Cauliflower Bake.

Turkey Patties

Ingredients

Turkey pieces – cooked

2 onions

2 to 3 large potatoes

Salt and pepper to taste

A dash of garlic paste and ginger paste.

A good dash of dried mixed herbs

2 eggs

Method

Mince turkey pieces

Slice onions

Dice and boil potatoes

Beat eggs

Mix the ingredients in a large bowl or a food processor.

Make into balls. Flatten on a floured board. You can either arrange balls on a tray and bake in the oven at 180°C (360°F), or fry in shallow oil.

Tips

Serve with a potato salad and a side salad.

Eat slowly, so you enjoy your food.

Remember your portion control

You can freeze the remaining patties for about a week.

Lamb Kebabs

Ingredients

Cooked lamb cut into cubes

Sliced mushrooms

Sliced red peppers (Capsicums)

Sliced Yellow peppers (Capsicums)

Cherry tomatoes

Onions cut into cubes

Soy Sauce

Balsamic vinegar

Dijon Mustard

Dash of ginger and garlic

Salt to taste

Method

Put all the ingredients into a bowl, mix well.

If you are using wooden skewers, soak them in water in a flat bowl for about ½ hour so they don't burn.

Start threading the kebab with a piece of lamb, mushroom, pepper, onion and cherry tomatoes until the skewers are full

Cook in a large flat frying pan or barbeque. Baste the kebabs with the remaining marinade.

Tips

Eat slowly, so you enjoy your food.

Remember your portion control

Pork stir-fry

Ingredients

Cooked pork

1 cup frozen peas

1 cup frozen corn

2 onions

Oil for frying onions

Curry leaves, Lemongrass, and pandanus leaf if available.

4 to 5 eggs

Salt & Pepper

Oyster sauce

Worcestershire sauce

Cooked rice

Roast potatoes (optional)

Sliced mushrooms (optional)

Method

Dice the pork

Beat the eggs, seasoned with salt, pepper and the sauces, and make an omelette. Cut the omelette up into pieces.

If the rice is cold heat it up with the Curry leaves, Lemongrass, and pandanus leaf if available.

Slice and fry the onions

Slice and fry the mushrooms

Cut roast potatoes

Cook the peas and corn in a little water in the microwave or on stove-top. Drain.

Put all ingredients in a large frying pan with a little heated oil.

Stir and cook for a few minutes until well heated through.

Tips

Eat slowly, so you enjoy your food.

Remember your portion control

Ham and Egg Cauliflower Bake

Ingredients

Cooked ham

½ cup oil

1 large onion

2 cups firm mushrooms

2 cups grated cheese

1 cauliflower

1 egg per person

Salt and pepper to taste.

Method

Slice the onion and mushrooms

Hard boil the eggs

Mash the cauliflower

Put the cauliflower in a pan with a little water to cover. Bring to the boil.

Cover pan and boil cauliflower for 1 minute. Drain.

Fry sliced onions

Mix onions, mushrooms, cauliflower, and half the cheese in an ovenproof dish and season.

Bury the eggs in the mixture spreading them out evenly. Make sure they are covered.

Sprinkle remaining cheese on top.

Bake in an oven at 180°C (360°F) for 20 minutes until the cheese on top starts to brown.

Tips

Eat slowly, so you enjoy your food.

Remember your portion control

www.ingramcontent.com/pod-product-compliance
Lightning Source LLC
Chambersburg PA
CBHW042015090526
44587CB00028B/4275